THE MUST-HAVE SLOW COOKBOOK

COOKBOOK

Simple Slow Cooker Recipes That Make Cooking Extra-Easy

Lovely Kitchen

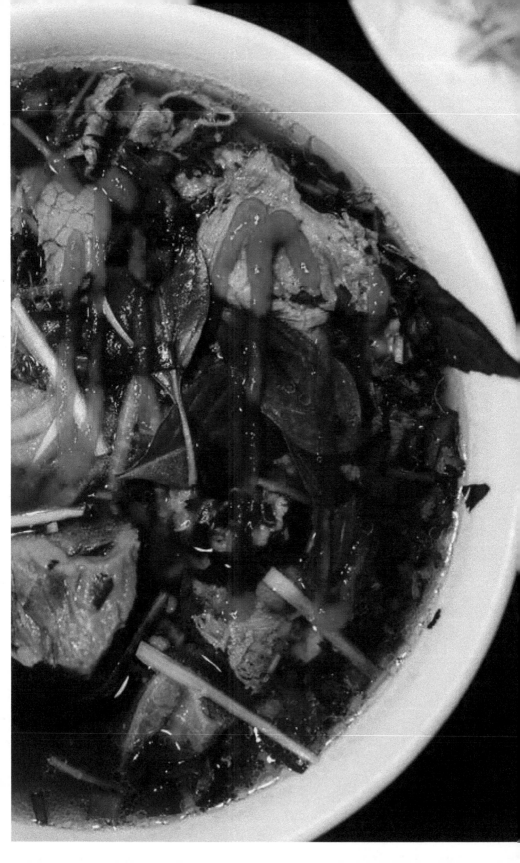

inattention, use, or misuse of the information in question by the reader will render any resulting actions solely under their purview. There are no scenarios in which the publisher or the original author of this work can be in any fashion deemed liable for any hardship or damages that may befall them after undertaking the information described herein.

Additionally, the information in the following pages is intended only for informational purposes and should thus be thought of as universal. As befitting its nature, it is presented without assurance regarding its prolonged validity or interim quality. Trademarks that are mentioned are done without written consent and can in no way be considered an endorsement from the trademark holder.

Table of Contents

INTRODUCTION 1

BREAKFAST 10

    Chocolate Toast 12

    Breakfast Casserole 14

    Light Egg Scramble.............................15

    Milk Oatmeal 17

    Butternut Squash Pate...........................18

    Strawberry Yogurt................................19

    Chocolate Oatmeal 20

    Zucchini Quinoa 22

    Apple Crumble 23

    Morning Pie.......................................24

LUNCH 26

Crock Pot Pizza 28

Savory Chowder 31

Carne Adovada 32

Bacon Swiss Pork Chops 33

Beef Stroganoff 34

Baked Chicken with Summer Vegetables 36

Beef Shwarma 38

Easy Chicken Curry 40

Beef and Bean Topped Baked Potatoes.............. 41

Chicken Philly Sandwiches 42

DINNER.. 45

Slow Cooker Pot Roast with Carrots and Shallots 47

Ultimate Slow Cooker Pot Roast 49

Easy Slow Cooker Pot Roast 51

Easy Fall-Apart Crock Pot Roast 53

The Best Crock Pot Roast 55

Chicken with Garlic and Mushrooms....................57

Chicken Verde with Peppers..............................59

Garlic Thyme Chicken 61

Greek-Style Chicken with White Beans 63

Sweet & Spicy Chicken.......................................65

Soy-Free Teriyaki Chicken & Veggies...................67

Easy Chicken Continental...................................70

DESSERT..72

Mediterranean Slow Cooker Apple Olive Cake 74

Mediterranean Crockpot Strawberry Basil Cobbler76

Slow Cooker Mediterranean Pumpkin Pecan Bread Pudding
....78

Slow Cooker Chocolate Fondue..........................80

Chocolate Orange Volcano Pudding....................82

Slow Cooker Nutella Fudge.................................84

Greek Yogurt Chocolate Mousse 87

Peanut Butter Banana Greek Yogurt Bowl........... 90

Italian Slow Cooker Banana Foster 93

Melon Pudding 94

Stuffed Peaches... 95

Sponge Cake 96

Semolina Pie.. 98

SOUP AND STEW 99

Fennel Stew... 101

Cabbage Stew.. 103

Smoked Sausage Stew...................................... 104

Meat Baby Carrot Stew 105

Jamaican Stew 106

INTRODUCTION

For many, cooking is more than a duty—it's a passion. Everyone wants healthy and delicious meals; however, our busy live soften don't leave much time for it.

A slow cooker is the perfect solution. It can easily handle both complicated and simple recipes, while eliminating the need to spend hours in the kitchen.

The slow cooker can cook almost all your favorite meals but in a healthier way. The most popular ingredients to use in the slow cooker are:

- meat and poultry
- fish
- vegetables
- soups
- oatmeal
- jams
- broths
- desserts

Keep in mind that the process has to be started long before eating time. Do the preparation in the morning and you can forget about cooking for the rest of the day. With the recipes in this cookbook, you will always have great ideas and delicious dinners ready for your family.

The slow cooker is easy to use and doesn't require professional cooking skills. It's easy enough for anyone, including busy moms, rushing professionals, teenagers, etc.

It is truly the easiest way to make a home-cooked meal. The hull of the slow cooker is made of stainless steel with a ceramic bowl inside so that the food doesn't burn. Simply add the food and cover it. Then select the desired cooking mode, normal or high, and set the time. Then you can go about your day. The slow cooker will sound a signal and automatically turn off when the timer runs out. At any point you can open the lid to add ingredients, and since the lid is made of heat-resistant glass, you can easily monitor the process.

Slow cookers come with either a sensor screen or buttons. Both are very easy to use. Cleaning the slow cooker is a simple process. The ceramic bowl is non-stick wipes clean very easily. The bowl and lid can be washed in a dish washer or by hand with a sponge.

It is safe to say that the slow cooker has more positive aspects than negative ones. One feature to watch for is whether the cord is long enough for where you want to put it. A few older models may not have a timer, which adds to the convenience.

However, once you get comfortable with your slow cooker, you will find it an indispensable tool in the kitchen. Let's sum up the advantages:

- Very little preparation required, leaving you plenty of time for other things
- Your food won't boil over or spill
- Makes great baby food
- Doesn't destroy the vitamins or flavor of the food
- Suitable for cooking broths, condensed milk, jams, and preserves

The slow cooker combines the best aspects of the oven and the stovetop. You can cook in it for many hours and still have a succulent and tender meal. It supports a healthy lifestyle and helps with special diets. It is also great for making baby food or dessert. As you can see, it is perfect for everyone!

A slow cooker will be an indispensable asset in your kitchen, and this cookbook will help you to impress your family with a vast variety of delicious and nutritious meals.

Choose the Right Slow Cooker for You

1. Size

Probably the most important consideration when buying your slow cooker is the size. Since a slow cooker works best when it's at least half full, it's important to think carefully about how much food you will want to prepare at a time.

Slow cookers come in a variety of sizes, from mini pots for dips to large pots for large families with plenty of options in between.

If you are single or a family of two, a two- to three-quart option is probably the best. If you have a family of three or four, the right size for you is probably a five-quart. Families of five or more will likely need six quarts or larger.

2. Shape

Another slow cooker parameter to consider is the shape. Slow cookers come in two basic shapes: round and oval. Round slow cookers are great for soups, stews, and chili peppers.

Ovals have a larger surface area, so there is more room for foods like pork chops and stuffed peppers. And because they have more surface area, they cook food a little faster than round slow cookers.

3. Cleaning

Each part should be easy to clean. A stainless steel exterior may show fingerprints and require additional cleaning.

4. Timer

A timer is useful because it alerts you when cooking is done and turns off the cooking process. Do not confuse this with a delayed start timer, which can turn the machine on while you are away.

5. Automatic Adjustment

This setting is useful because it will bring the food to a high temperature and then switch to low for the remaining cooking time.

Top Tips for the Slow Cooker

1. Cut down cooking time by preparing ingredients in advance

Most of the ingredients for a slow cooker can be prepared (cut, peeled, chopped, diced) in advance. Put all prepared ingredients in a Ziploc bag and store it in the fridge. This will preserve the vital minerals and vitamins of the products and speed up the process of starting the meal.

2. Use fat from the meat instead of using additional fats and oils

Cut the fat from the meat and put it in the bottom of the slow cooker. Then add all of the remaining ingredients. This will help avoid overcooking and reduce the amount of needed oil.

3. Get rid of extra liquid

Sometimes you cannot calculate the amount of liquid you need. There is a trick that will help you easily reduce soupiness: mix one tablespoon of flour with three tablespoons of water and whisk it until smooth. Then add the liquid to the pot during cooking and stir well. In a few minutes, the excess liquid will thicken up. If this trick doesn't work, add more flour or mix it with cornstarch.

4. Save time by adding all ingredients at once

Often, slow cooker recipes recommend adding the ingredients at different times; however, it is usually fine to add all components at once. Bear in mind that meats and vegetables often require different cooking times.

5. More time for achieving the perfect taste

Some meals such as stews, soups, ragout, oatmeal, and pies taste better after they've rested for a while. Leave the finished dish for 4-5 hours or overnight and you will taste the difference.

6. Crockpot liners

Liners are a great solution for those who hate cleaning the slow cooker after cooking. Put it over the slow cooker bowl and then close the lid. This will eliminate the need to scrub off any stuck pieces.

7. Add milk at the end of cooking

Milk has a tendency to curdle while cooking. Furthermore, it can cause high foam while boiling. That is why it is recommended to add milk at the end of the cooking process or mix it with water.

8. Open the lid only when the meal is cooked

Once you have added all the ingredients, do not reopen the lid of the slow cooker unless the instructions call for stirring or removing certain ingredients. The slow cooker lid retains the heat, and after being opened, it will take some time to reach the proper cooking temperature again.

9. Cheap cuts of meat are the best

Use the cheap cuts of meat such as brisket, chuck, shoulder, etc. They will take a longer cooking time, but the miracle of the slow cooker is that even the toughest cuts of meat will end up wonderfully tender and succulent.

10. Increase or decrease the cooking time manually

If you need to speed up cooking time, the special conversion will help you to make the correct adjustments.

BREAKFAST

Chocolate Toast

4 Servings

Preparation time: 55 minutes

Ingredients

- 1 banana, mashed
- 1 tablespoon coconut oil
- ¼ cup full-fat milk
- 4 white bread slices
- 1 tablespoon vanilla extract
- 2 tablespoons Nutella

Direction

- Mix vanilla extract, Nutella, mashed banana, coconut oil, and milk.
- Pour the mixture in the slow cooker and cook on High for 40 minutes.
- Make a quick pressure release and cool the chocolate mixture.
- Spread the toasts with a cooked mixture.

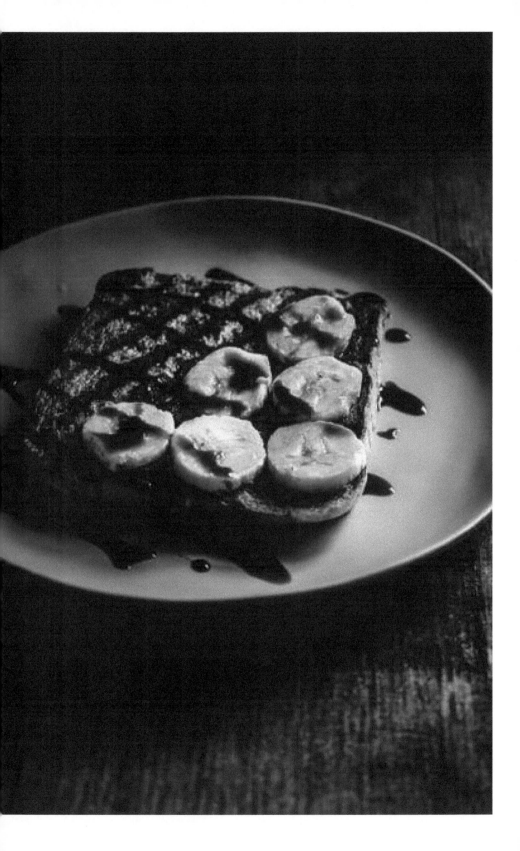

Breakfast Casserole

5 Servings

Preparation time: 7 hours 15 minutes

Ingredients

- ½ teaspoon cayenne pepper
- 5 eggs, beaten
- 5 oz ham, chopped
- ½ cup bell pepper, chopped
- 1 cup Cheddar cheese, shredded
- 1 potato, peeled, diced
- ½ cup carrot, grated
- 1 teaspoon ground turmeric

Direction

- Make the layer from potato in the slow cooker mold.
- Then put the layer of carrot over the potatoes.
- Sprinkle the vegetables with ground turmeric and cayenne pepper.
- Then add ham and bell pepper.
- Pour the beaten eggs over the casserole and top with shredded cheese.
- Cook the meal on LOW for 7 hours.

Light Egg Scramble

2 Servings

Preparation time: 15 minutes 4 hours

Ingredients

- 1 tablespoon butter, melted
- 1 teaspoon salt
- 1 teaspoon ground paprika
- 6 eggs, beaten

Direction

- Pour the melted butter into the slow cooker.
- Add eggs and salt and stir.
- Cook the eggs on Low for 4 hours. Stir the eggs every 15 minutes.
- When the egg scramble is cooked, top it with ground paprika.

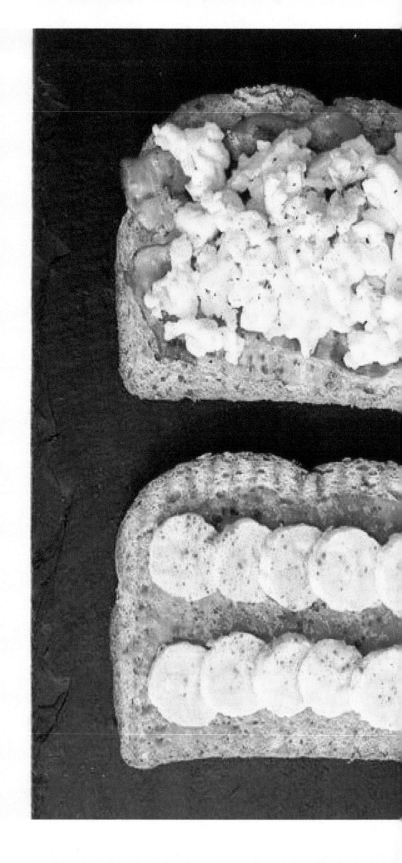

Milk Oatmeal

4 Servings

Preparation time: 10 minutes, 2 hours

Ingredients

- Liquid honey
- 1 teaspoon vanilla extract
- 1 tablespoon coconut oil
- ¼ teaspoon ground cinnamon
- 2 cups oatmeal
- 1 cup of water
- 1 cup milk
- 1 tablespoon

Direction

- Put all ingredients except liquid honey in the slow cooker and mix.
- Close the lid and cook the meal on High for 2 hours.
- Then stir the cooked oatmeal and transfer it into the serving bowls.
- Top the meal with a small amount of liquid honey.

Butternut Squash Pate

7 Servings

Preparation time: 7 minutes, 4 hours

Ingredients

- ¼ teaspoon ground clove
- 1 tablespoon lemon juice
- 2 tablespoons coconut oil
- 8 oz butternut squash puree
- 1 tablespoon honey
- 1 teaspoon cinnamon

Direction

- Put all ingredients in the slow cooker, gently stir, and cook on Low for 4 hours.

Strawberry Yogurt

7 Servings

Preparation time: 15 hours 3 hours

Ingredients

- 1 cup strawberries, sliced
- 1 teaspoon coconut shred
- 4 cups milk
- 1 cup Greek yogurt

Direction

- Pour the milk into the slow cooker and cook it on HIGH for 3 hours.
- Cool the milk till it reaches the temperature of 100F.
- Add Greek yogurt, mix the liquid carefully, and cover with a towel.
- Leave the yogurt for 10 hours in a warm place.
- Pour the thick yogurt mixture into the colander or cheese mold and leave for 5 hours to avoid the extra liquid.
- Transfer the cooked yogurt into the ramekins and top with sliced strawberries and coconut shred.

Chocolate Oatmeal

5 Servings

Preparation time: 10 minutes, 4 hours

Ingredients

- 2 cups oatmeal
- ½ teaspoon ground cardamom
- 1 oz dark chocolate, chopped
- 1 teaspoon vanilla extract
- 2 cups of coconut milk

Direction

- Put all ingredients in the slow cooker and stir carefully with the help of the spoon.
- Close the lid and cook the meal for 4 hours on Low.

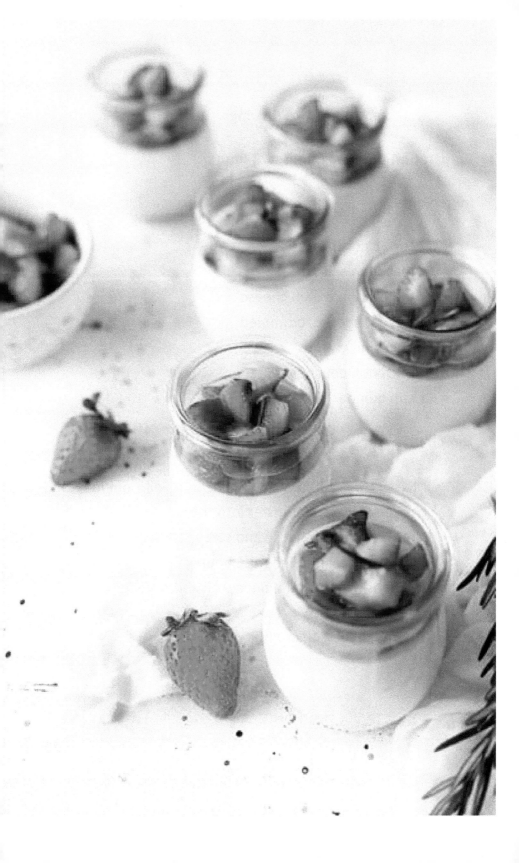

Zucchini Quinoa

3 Servings

Preparation time: 10 minutes, 3 hours

Ingredients

- 2 cups chicken stock
- 1 teaspoon salt
- 1 tablespoon cream cheese
- 1 oz goat cheese, crumbled
- ½ zucchini, grated
- 1 teaspoon coconut oil
- 1 cup quinoa

Direction

- Mix grated zucchini with coconut oil, quinoa, and chicken stock and transfer into the slow cooker.
- Then add cream cheese and salt.
- Cook the meal on High for 3 hours.
- Then stir the cooked quinoa well and transfer it into the serving plates.
- Top the meal with crumbled goat cheese.

Apple Crumble

2 Servings

Preparation time: 10 minutes, 5 hours

Ingredients

- 4 tablespoons water
- 1 tablespoon almond butter
- 1 teaspoon vanilla extract
- 1 tablespoon liquid honey
- 2 Granny Smith apples
- 4 oz granola

Direction

- Cut the apple into small wedges.
- Remove the seeds from the apples and chop them into small pieces.
- Put them in the slow cooker.
- Add water, almond butter, vanilla extract, and honey.
- Cook the apples for 5 hours on Low.
- Then stir them carefully.
- Put the cooked apples and granola one by one in the serving glasses.

Morning Pie

6 Servings

Preparation time: 10 minutes hours

Ingredients

- 1 teaspoon vanilla extract
- ½ teaspoon ground cinnamon
- 1 teaspoon sesame oil
- 4 pecans, crushed
- ½ cup oatmeal
- 1 cups full-fat milk
- 1 cup butternut squash, diced

Direction

- Mix oatmeal and milk in the slow cooker.
- Add diced butternut squash, vanilla extract, and ground cinnamon.
- Then add sesame oil and pecans.
- Carefully mix the ingredients and close the lid.
- Cook the pie on Low for 3 hours.
- Then cool the pie and cut it into servings.

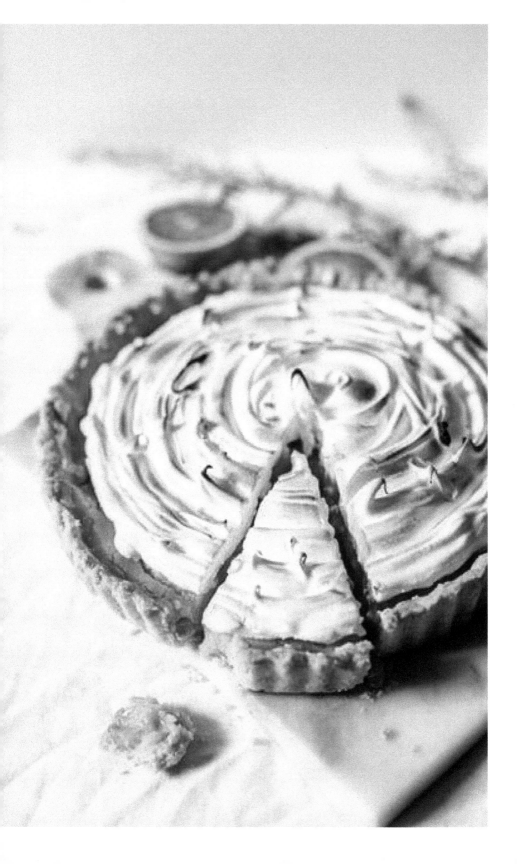

LUNCH

Crock Pot Pizza

6 Servings

Preparation Time: 5 hours 15 minutes

Ingredients

- ¾ pound ground Beef, cooked
- 1 (15 ounces) jar Pizza sauce
- 3 cups fresh Spinach
- 16 Pepperoni slices
- 1 cup Mushrooms, sliced
- ½ cup sweet Onion, chopped
- ¾ pound Italian sausage, cooked
- 3 cups Mozzarella cheese, shredded
- 1 cup Olives, sliced
- ¼ cup sun-dried Tomatoes, chopped
- ½ green pepper, chopped
- ¼ cup marinated Artichoke hearts, chopped
- 2 Garlic cloves, minced

Directions

- Mix together sausage and ground beef with onions and sauce.
- Place half of the sauce mixture in the crockpot and layer with half of the spinach.

28

- Arrange pepperoni on the spinach and top with half of the remaining ingredients ending with mozzarella cheese.
- Repeat the layering and cover the lid of the crockpot.
- Cook on Low for about 5 hours and dish out.

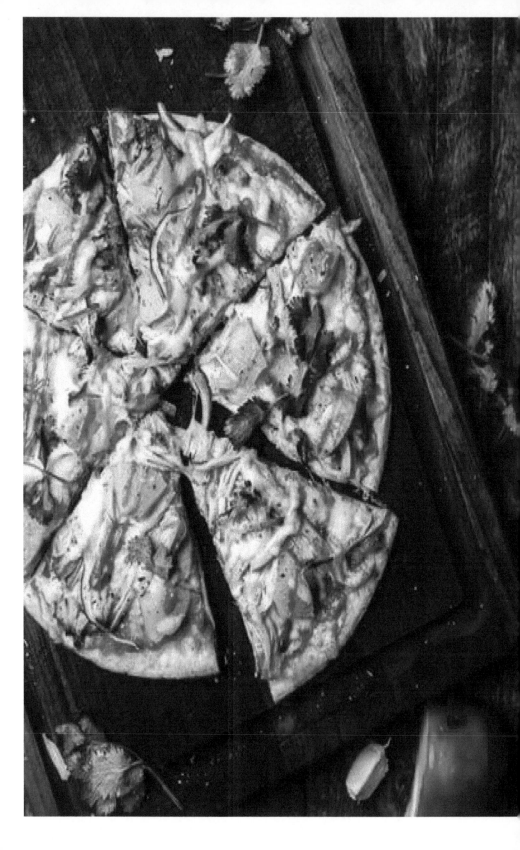

Savory Chowder

8 Servings

Preparation Time: 6 hours 20 minutes

Ingredients

- 1 can clams
- 1 cup organic Chicken broth
- 1 pint Half-and-half
- 2 slices bacon, cooked
- 1 teaspoon salt
- ¼ cup red Onions, chopped
- 2 cups cauliflower, chopped
- ¼ teaspoon Thyme
- 2 teaspoons Parsley
- 1 Garlic clove, minced
- 1/8 teaspoon Pepper

Directions

- Put all the ingredients in a crockpot and stir well.
- Cover and cook on LOW for about 6 hours.
- Ladle out in a bowl and serve hot.

Carne Adovada

8 Servings

Preparation Time: 6 hours 20 minutes

Ingredients

- 1 teaspoon ground Cumin
- 3 cups Chicken broth
- 2 Garlic cloves, minced
- ½ teaspoon Salt
- 1/8 cup Canola oil
- 12 hot New Mexico red chili pods
- 2 pounds boneless Pork shoulder, chunked
- 1 teaspoon Mexican oregano

Directions

- Put canola oil and pork shoulder in a pan over medium heat and cook for about 2 minutes on each side.
- Transfer to a crockpot and stir in the remaining ingredients.
- Cover and cook on Low for about 6 hours.
- Dish out and serve hot.

Bacon Swiss Pork Chops

6 Servings

Preparation Time: 8 hours 10 minutes

Ingredients

- 8 Pork chops, bone-in
- 2 tablespoons Butter
- Salt and Black pepper, to taste
- 12 Bacon strips, cut in half
- 1 cup Swiss Cheese, shredded

Direction

- Season the pork chops with salt and black pepper.
- Put the butter, seasoned pork chops and shredded Swiss cheese in the crockpot.
- Cover and cook on Low for about 7 hours.
- Stir in the cheese mixture and cook on Low for 1 more hour.

Beef Stroganoff

8 Servings

Preparation Time: 8 hours 25 minutes

Ingredients

- ¼ teaspoon G-salt
- 1½ cups Beef bouillon
- 2 pounds round Steak
- 1/8 teaspoon Black pepper
- 1 teaspoon Salt
- ½ pound fresh Mushrooms
- 1 cup Sour cream

Directions

- Season steaks with salt and black pepper.
- Place the seasoned steaks, garlic salt and beef bouillon in the crockpot.
- Cover and cook on Low for about 8 hours.
- Add in fresh mushrooms and sour cream.
- Cover it and cook on High for about 15 minutes.
- Dish out and serve hot.

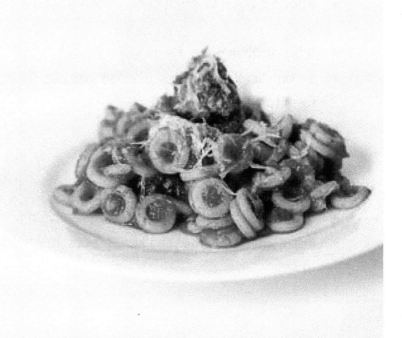

Baked Chicken with Summer Vegetables

6 Servings

Preparation Time: 5 Hours

Ingredients

- 2 Tbs. dijon Mustard
- Salt and Pepper
- 1 tsp. Thyme
- 1 Onion cut in thick wedges
- 4 large cloves Garlic minced
- Red bell pepper sliced
- Green bell pepper sliced
- About 3 pounds of chicken I used a whole chicken, cut up
- A bit of Olive oil
- 1 can diced Tomatoes drained (or use fresh, chopped tomatoes)
- 1/2 cup white Wine

Directions

- Rub the inside of the crockpot with olive oil.
- Rinse and pat the chicken pieces dry with a paper towel.

- Rub the undersides of the chicken with dijon mustard and sprinkle with salt, pepper and thyme. Place them in the bottom of the crockpot, skin side down.
- Put the veggies and wine on top of the chicken.
- Cover and bake on high for 5 hours or so. Or bake on low 7-8 hours.
- Serve with angel hair pasta or baked potatoes.

Beef Shwarma

6 Servings

Preparation Time: 7 Hours

Ingredients

- 2 dashes ground Red pepper
- 3 Garlic cloves crushed
- 2.5 - 3 lbs. thin cut boneless Beef steak
- 8 oz plain or Greek yogurt
- 6 Tbs. Lemon juice
- 6 Tbs. Olive oil
- 1 tsp. Salt
- 2 tsps. Curry powder
- 1 small Cucumber chopped
- Pita bread

Directions

- Stir lemon juice, olive oil, salt, curry, cayenne pepper and garlic together in a small bowl.
- Place meat in slow cooker.
- Pour mixture over the top and stir to combine with meat.
- Cook on high 5-6 hours or low 7-8 hours

- Combine yogurt and cucumber.
- Serve cooked meat in pita bread with cucumber-yogurt sauce.

Easy Chicken Curry

8 Servings

Preparation Time: 7 Hours

Ingredients

- 1 cup Salsa
- 3 Tbs. Curry powder
- 1 can Coconut milk
- 3 lbs. boneless Chicken
- 1 Onion chopped
- 2 cups Rice cooked

Directions

- Place chicken, onion, salsa and curry powder in slow cooker.
- Cook on high 5-6 hours or low 7-8 hours.
- Minutes before serving remove chicken from slow cooker.
- Add in coconut milk to slow cooker. Stir into sauce.
- Return chicken to pot.
- Serve over cooked rice.

Beef and Bean Topped Baked Potatoes

8 Servings

Preparation Time: 7 Hours

Ingredients

- 1 Garlic clove pressed or minced
- 1 can kidney Beans rinsed and drained
- 1 can chili ready diced tomatoes
- Baking potatoes
- 1 lb. ground Beef cooked
- 1/2 cup Onion and Bacon cooked
- Shredded Cheddar cheese

Directions

- Place all the ingredients, except the potatoes and cheese in the slow cooker or heat them together on the stove.
- Top baked potatoes and sprinkle with shredded cheese, if desired.

Chicken Philly Sandwiches

7 Servings

Preparation Time: 8 Hours

Ingredients

- ¼ tsp. Paprika
- 1 large (or 2 small) Bell peppers, sliced
- 1 medium Onion, sliced
- 2 cups sliced Mushrooms
- Salt and Pepper to season the bell peppers, Onions, and Mushrooms
- 2 lbs. boneless skinless Chicken breasts
- 1 cup Chicken broth
- ¼ tsp. Salt
- ¼ tsp. Pepper
- ¼ tsp. Garlic powder
- French bread or hoagie rolls for servings
- Swiss cheese for serving (use reduced-fat)

Directions

- Place the chicken breasts into a 4-quart or larger slow cooker, and pour over the chicken broth. Season the chicken with the salt, pepper, garlic powder, and paprika.

- Cover and cook on Low for 6.5 hours.
- After the chicken has cooked, add the sliced vegetables on top of the cooked chicken.
- Cover and cook on high for 1.5 hours more.
- With 2 forks shred the chicken.
- Using tongs place the meat onto hoagies, and top with cheese. Place the sandwiches open-faced under the broiler in the oven to toast the buns and melt the cheese.

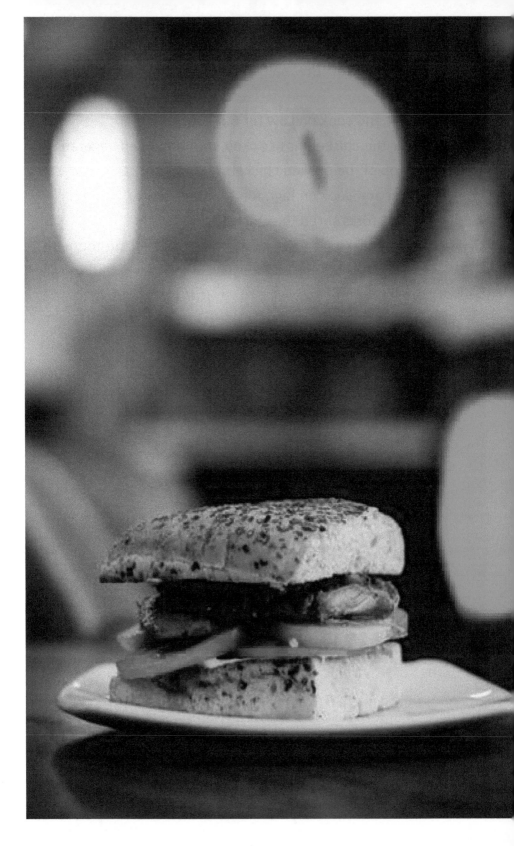

DINNER

Slow Cooker Pot Roast with Carrots and Shallots

8 Servings

Preparation Time: 6 Hours

Ingredients

- 14 baby Carrots peeled (or five large carrots cut into thirds)
- 8 Shallots peeled
- Sea Salt
- 1/2 cup Beef broth
- 3 lbs Chuck Roast
- 1/4 cup red Wine optional but gives a richer flavor
- Butter ghee or Coconut oil

Directions

- Generously season roast with sea salt, pepper, garlic powder and herbs de Provence. Heat a cast iron pan on med/high heat. When pan is hot add enough butter, ghee or coconut oil to lightly coat the bottom on the pan.
- Place roast in pan and brown the first side, turn over and brown the second side (usually about 4-5 minutes a side) then place meat in slow cooker, add broth and wine.

- Add shallots and carrots to crock pot, sprinkle with sea salt, freshly ground pepper and herbs de Provence. Place lid on crock pot and cook either 4 hours on high or 8 hours on low. Carve beef against the grain and serve.

Ultimate Slow Cooker Pot Roast

6 Servings

Preparation Time: 8 Hours

Ingredients

- 1 pound Carrots peeled and cut into 2" chunks
- 2 pounds Yukon Gold Potatoes peeled and cut into large chunks
- 2 cloves Garlic minced
- 2 cups Beef broth
- 2 tablespoons Corn starch
- 4-5 pound chuck Roast
- 2 tablespoons Canola oil
- 2 teaspoons Kosher salt
- 1 teaspoon coarse ground Black pepper
- 1 teaspoon dried Thyme
- 2 tablespoons cold Water
- Minced Parsley optional, to garnish

Directions

- Season the chuck roast with the Kosher salt, pepper and thyme (if you are sensitive to sodium, adjust to your taste or you can even leave the salt out altogether since you're adding broth).

49

- Heat your pan (or if you can brown in your slow cooker, do it in that insert to medium high.
- Add the canola oil and when it ripples and is hot add in the roast and brown, deeply, for 4-5 minutes on each side.
- In your slow cooker add the carrots, potatoes and garlic.
- Lay the beef on top, then add the beef broth and cover, cooking on low for 8-10 hours or on high for 5-6 hours.
- In the last hour mix your cornstarch and water and add it to the slow cooker to thicken the sauce or you can take the food out when done cooking, and add the leftover liquid to a small saucepan with the cornstarch/water mixture and cook on high for just 2-3 minutes until the liquid is thickened into a gravy.
- Pour the gravy over the meat and garnish with parsley if desired.

Easy Slow Cooker Pot Roast

8 Servings

Preparation Time: 4 Hours

Ingredients

- 8 cloves Garlic smashed with the back of a spoon (or 2 tablespoons minced garlic)
- 1 pound (500 grams) baby Potatoes, white or Yukon gold, (you may need to halve them if they are too large)
- 4 large Carrots, cut into 2-inch pieces
- 2 stalks Celery, cut into 1-inch pieces
- 1/4 cup Balsamic vinegar
- 1 tablespoon Olive oil
- 4 pounds (2 kg) chuck Roast or blade roast, boneless and trimmed of excess fat
- 2 yellow Onions chopped
- 2 tablespoons Dijon Mustard
- 1 tablespoon Brown sugar
- 2 teaspoons dried Thyme
- 1-2 teaspoons Vgetable stock powder or bullion powder
- 1 teaspoon salt, or to taste
- 1/2 teaspoon freshly ground Black pepper, or to taste
- 1 cup reduced-sodium Beef broth
- 2 tablespoons plain Flour (optional -- for a thick gravy)
- 2 tablespoons fresh chopped Parsley, to serve

Directions

- Heat oil in a large skillet or pan over high heat. Season roast with a good amount of salt and pepper. Sear on all sides until browned (about 5-6 minutes each side). Transfer roast to the bowl of a 6-quart slow cooker.
- Add the onions, garlic, potatoes, carrots, celery, vinegar, mustard, brown sugar, thyme, stock powder and salt and pepper to taste. Mix the stock together with the flour and pour into the slow cooker bowl
- Cook on high setting for 4-5 hours, or low for 6-8 hours, OR until meat is tender and falling apart, and the vegetables are soft.
- Taste test and add any extra balsamic vinegar, brown sugar, salt or pepper, until reaching your desired flavour.
- Slice beef. Garnish with parsley, drizzle over the gravy and sprinkle with black cracked pepper to serve! ENJOY!

Easy Fall-Apart Crock Pot Roast

6 Servings

Preparation Time: 8 Hours

Ingredients

- 5 Garlic cloves, peeled and smashed
- 5 Carrots, peeled and cut into 2.5cm/1" pieces
- 3 Celery stalks, cut into 4 cm / 1.5" pieces
- 1 cup / 250 ml dry red Wine (or sub with beef broth)
- 3 cups / 750 ml Beef broth, salt reduced
- 1/3 cup / 50g Flour (plain / all purpose)
- 1 tsp dried Rosemary
- 1 ½ tsps dried Thyme
- 1 - 2 kg / 2 - 4 lb Beef chuck roast / rolled chuck
- Salt and Pepper
- 2 tbsps Olive oil
- 1 Onion (large), cut into large dice
- 750 g - 1 kg / 1.5 - 2 lb Potatoes, peeled and cut into 2.5 cm / 1" pieces

Directions

- Pat beef dry with paper towels. Sprinkle generously with salt and pepper all over.

- Heat oil in a pan over high heat. Brown aggressively all over - a deep dark brown crust is essential for flavour base! Should take about 7 minutes.
- Transfer beef to slow cooker.
- In the same pan, add onion and garlic. Cook for 2 minutes until onion is browned.
- Add wine, reduce by half. Transfer to slow cooker.
- Mix together flour and about 1 cup of the broth. Lumps are fine. Pour into slow cooker.
- Add remaining broth, carrots, celery, rosemary and thyme into slow cooker.
- Cover and slow cook on low for 5 hours. Or 45 minutes in a pressure cook on high.
- Add potato, slow cook on low for 3 hours. Or 10 minutes in a pressure cooker on high.
- Remove beef. Rest for 5 minutes, then slice thickly.
- Adjust salt and pepper of Sauce to taste. Serve beef with vegetables and plenty of sauce!

The Best Crock Pot Roast

8 Servings

Preparation Time: 8 Hours

Ingredients

- 1 teaspoon Paprika
- ½ teaspoon dried Thyme
- 1 teaspoon dried Rosemary
- 2 tablespoons Olive oil
- 1 large yellow Onion cut into large pieces
- 2 pounds russet Potatoes peeled and cut into 2-inch chunks
- 1 pound Carrots peeled and cut into 2-inch pieces
- 2 cloves Garlic minced
- 2 cups Beef broth or stock
- 2-3 pound chuck Roast
- 1 ½ teaspoons Salt
- ½ teaspoon Black pepper
- 1 teaspoon Garlic powder
- 2 tablespoons Cornstarch
- 2 tablespoons Water
- Fresh minced Parsley

Directions

- Rinse the roast and pat it dry. Mix salt, pepper, garlic powder, paprika, thyme and rosemary and rub into the roast on all sides.
- Heat olive oil in a large skillet over a medium heat. Brown roast on all sides; about 3-4 minutes per side.
- Place carrots, onion, garlic and potatoes into the slow cooker. Pour in beef broth, then set the browned chuck roast on top.
- Cover and cook on low 8-10 hours or on high for 5-6 hours.
- Transfer the meat and vegetables to a serving dish. Combine water and cornstarch in a small bowl then pour into the slow cooker. Whisk together to combine. Cover and cook on high for 5 minutes, just enough to thicken the gravy.
- Serve meat and vegetables smothered in gravy, with minced parsley for garnish if desired.

Chicken with Garlic and Mushrooms

8 Servings

Preparation Time: 7 hours 10 minutes

Ingredients

- 10 Garlic cloves
- 2 pounds Chicken thighs
- 1 cup Mushrooms, sliced
- 2 tablespoons Butter
- Salt and Black pepper, to taste

Directions

- Season the chicken thighs with salt and black pepper.
- Put the butter, garlic, mushrooms and seasoned chicken in the crockpot.
- Cover and cook on Low for about 7 hours.
- Dish out and serve hot.

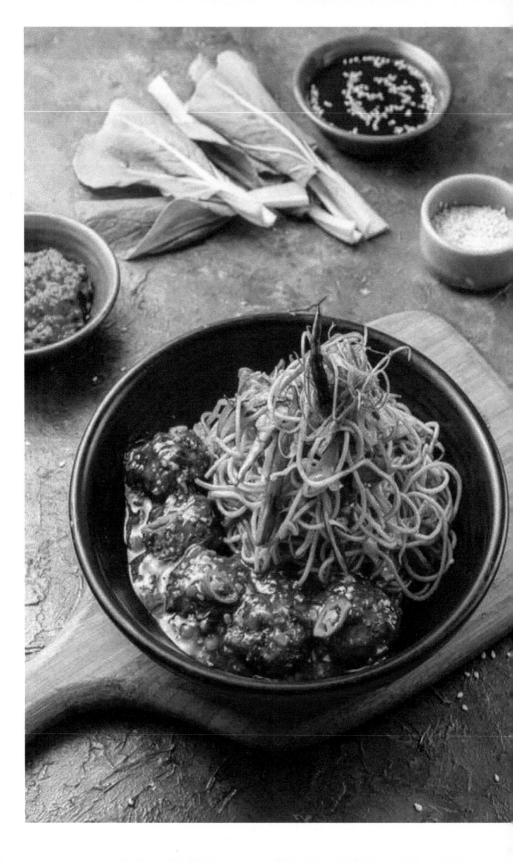

Chicken Verde with Peppers

7 Servings

Preparation Time: 7 Hours

Ingredients

- 1 1/2 tsps Sea salt
- 1 tsp Garlic powder
- 1/2 tsp Paprika
- 1/4 tsp Cumin
- 1 (12oz) jar Salsa Verde
- 1 large sweet Onion
- lbs boneless, skinless Chicken thighs
- 2 red Bell peppers (or use a combination of red and yellow peppers)
- Optional: Bibb lettuce leaves to make wraps

Directions

- Cut the ends off of the onion and then slice into five thick slices. Place in the bottom of a 6-quart slow cooker.
- Place the chicken thighs on top of the onion. In a small bowl, combine the seasonings and evenly distribute the seasoning mix across the top of the chicken.

- Then, evenly spoon the jar of salsa verde over the top of the seasoned chicken.
- Slice the red bell peppers into thick slices; discard the seeds and stem. You can either - place the sliced pepper over the salsa and cook with the chicken for very soft pepper slices – or add the sliced peppers during the last hour of cook time to enjoy them al dente.
- Cover and cook on high 5-6 hours or on low 7-8 hours.
- When chicken is done, use a slotted spoon to move the peppers to the side and carefully remove just the chicken and place it on a large platter. Use two forks to shred the chicken.
- Remove the pepper and onion slices and place on a serving plate.
- Serve the chicken & veggies with large Bibb lettuce leaves to make lettuce wraps. Top with your favorite fajita toppings, such as pico de gallo, diced avocado, fresh minced cilantro, etc. Enjoy!

Garlic Thyme Chicken

8 Servings

Preparation Time: 7 Hours

Ingredients

- 3 lbs bone-in Chicken thighs
- 1 tbsp Olive oil
- 20 Garlic cloves (about 2 large heads of garlic)
- 2 tsps Sea salt
- 1 tsp dried Thyme
- 1 large sweet Onion, peeled and sliced into thin rings
- 1 tsp Paprika
- 1 tsp fresh-ground Black pepper

Directions

- In the bottom of a 6-quart slow cooker, evenly distribute the sliced onion along the bottom.
- Smash and peel the garlic cloves, making sure to gather 15-20 large cloves. (See note below on "how to smash garlic," if you're unfamiliar with this method.)
- Place the chicken thighs into a large mixing bowl and drizzle with olive oil. Add the smashed garlic cloves and toss to combine.

- Sprinkle the seasonings across the top of the chicken-garlic mixture and toss until chicken is well coated with seasonings.
- Transfer the chicken-garlic mixture to the slow cooker and cover.
- Cook on low for 6-7 hours, or on high for 4-5 hours. Serve with a vegetables.

Greek-Style Chicken with White Beans

8 Servings

Preparation Time: 7 Hours

Ingredients

- 2 tbsps Lemon juice (approx. 1 lemon)
- 15 oz. fire-roasted Tomatoes, diced
- 1/2 cup pitted Kalamata olives, halved
- 2 cups soaked & cooked White beans
- Optional: Lemon slices and crumbled goat cheese for serving
- Greek Seasoning Mix
- 1 large yellow Onion, chopped
- 3 cloves of Garlic, crushed and sliced
- 3 lbs. bone-in Chicken thighs, skin removed
- 1 tsp dried Oregano
- 1/2 tsp each of Onion powder, Garlic powder, Parsley, Thyme and Sea salt
- 1/4 tsp freshly ground Black pepper
- Pinch of Nutmeg

Directions

- Lightly coat the bottom of a 6-quart slow cooker with olive oil or coconut oil.

- In a small bowl, combine the Greek Seasoning Mix ingredients. Evenly distribute the seasoning mix among the chicken thighs by sprinkling both sides of each thigh with the seasoning mix.
- Place chopped onion and garlic in bottom of slow cooker. Then arrange the seasoned chicken thighs over the onions and drizzle the lemon juice across the top.
- Evenly spoon the tomatoes and olives on top of each chicken thigh.
- Cover and cook on high for 5-6 hours or on low for 7-8 hours.
- During the last 30 minutes of cooking time, carefully remove the chicken thighs (tongs work best) and place on a platter. Stir in the beans, if using – otherwise, skip this step. Then carefully add the chicken back to the crockpot and continue cooking.
- When ready to serve, place about a half-cup of rice on each plate, if desired. Then place the chicken thighs over the rice with a large ladle or two of the white bean mixture. Garnish with lemon wedges and crumbled goat cheese, if desired. Enjoy!

Sweet & Spicy Chicken

8 Servings

Preparation Time: 7 Hours

Ingredients

- 1 red Bell pepper, seeded and sliced
- 1 yellow Bell pepper, seeded and sliced
- 3 lbs boneless, skinless Chicken thighs
- 3 cups Broccoli florets
- For the sweet & spicy sauce
- 2 cloves Garlic, minced
- 2 Tbsps Coconut aminos
- 2 Tbsps dry Mustard
- 2 tsps dried minced Onion
- 2 tsps Sea salt
- 1/2 tsp ground Ginger
- 2 cups all-fruit Apricot jam
- 1/2 tsp red Pepper flakes (use more for a spicier sauce)
- 2 Tbsps arrowroot powder (for thickening sauce)

Directions

- Cut chicken thighs into bite-size chunks and place into a 6-quart slow cooker.

- Cut the vegetables as noted above. Place in a bowl and refrigerate until ready to use, as noted below.
- In a medium bowl, whisk together the apricot jam, garlic, soy sauce or coconut aminos, mustard, onion, salt, ginger, and red-pepper flakes. Pour over the chicken.
- Cover and cook on low for 4 to 5 hours. Check chicken at the 4-hour mark, if it's not cooked through, continue cooking. Once the chicken is cooked through, add the sliced bell peppers and broccoli florets. Then, continue cooking on low until vegetables are al dente (about 30-45 minutes).
- Use a slotted spoon to remove chicken and vegetables from the slow cooker and place in a serving dish. Whisk in the arrowroot powder to thicken the sauce, if desired.
- To serve, ladle the sauce over the chicken and vegetables. Serve over basmati rice.
- To Freeze: Place the vegetables into a freezer-safe container and freeze. Add the diced chicken to a separate freezer-safe container, top with the sweet-n-spicy sauce, and freeze.
- To Prepare: Thaw the chicken mixture and vegetables in the refrigerator overnight. When ready to cook, follow the instructions above beginning in Step 4. Easy and delicious!

Soy-Free Teriyaki Chicken & Veggies

8 Servings

Preparation Time: 7 Hours

Ingredients

Chicken

- lbs. boneless, skinless Chicken thighs
- 3-4 green Onions, plus more for topping
- Teriyaki Sauce
- 1 tablespoon rice Vinegar
- 2 cloves Garlic, minced
- 3/4 tsp Sea salt
- 1/2 tsp ground Ginger
- 1/2 tsp red Pepper flakes
- 1/2 cup all-fruit Apricot preserves
- 1/3 cup Coconut aminos (I use this in place of soy sauce)
- 2 tablespoons Honey
- 2 tsps Arrowroot powder (used to thicken sauce)
- Vegetables
- 2 cups Julienne carrots
- 4 cups fresh Broccoli florets
- 2 cups snap Peas

Directions

- Arrange the 3-4 stalks of green onion (a.k.a. scallions) along the bottom of a 6-quart slow cooker. Place the chicken on top of the green onions.
- In a small bowl, whisk together all of the teriyaki sauce ingredients EXCEPT the arrowroot powder, until well combined. Carefully spoon the sauce over the chicken.
- Cover and cook on high for 4-5 hours or on low 6-7 hours. During the last 1.5 to 2 hours of cook time, add the vegetables. Cover and continue cooking until vegetables are al dente (cook time for the vegetables may vary, especially if you're cooking on the low setting).
- Use a slotted spoon to remove the vegetables and chicken; transfer to a serving platter. Discard the green onion stalks.
- To make the Teriyaki Sauce: Pour the remaining liquid in the slow cooker through a fine-mesh strainer into a large measuring cup or bowl. Place 1 1/4 cups of the liquid into a small saucepan, discard the remainder.
- In a small prep bowl, add the 2 teaspoons of arrowroot powder and 2 tablespoons of water, mixing to create a slurry. Add the arrowroot mixture to the saucepan and whisk well to combine.
- Heat the teriyaki sauce over medium heat, whisking frequently until sauce thickens. Re-season to taste with

additional sea salt and ginger, if necessary. Transfer teriyaki sauce to a serving bowl.

- Spoon the teriyaki sauce over the chicken and vegetables. Then, top with a sprinkling of sliced fresh green onions, if desired. Enjoy!

Easy Chicken Continental

2 Servings

Preparation time: 15 minutes 7 hours

Ingredients

- ½ cup cream
- ½ can onion soup
- 2 oz dried beef
- 8 oz chicken breast, skinless, boneless, chopped
- 1 tablespoon cornstarch

Direction

- Put 1 oz of the dried beef in the slow cooker in one layer.
- Then add chicken breast and top it with remaining dried beef.
- After this, mix cream cheese, onion, and cornstarch. Whisk the mixture and pour it over the chicken and dried beef.
- Cook the meal on Low for 7 hours.

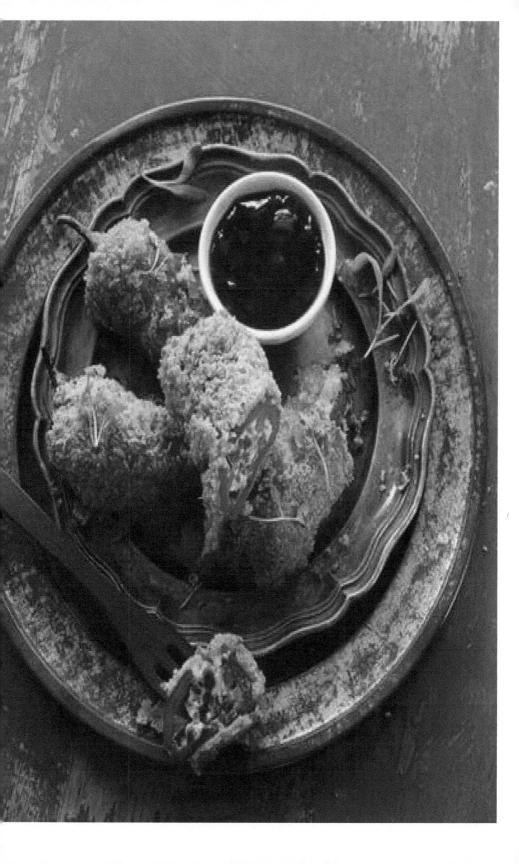

DESSERT

Mediterranean Slow Cooker Apple Olive Cake

6 Servings

Preparation Time: 2 hours 20 minutes

Ingredients

- 3 cups Whole wheat Flour
- 2 cups Orange juice
- 1 teaspoon Baking powder
- ½ teaspoon Ground nutmeg
- 1 cup Sugar
- 1 teaspoon Baking soda
- 3 Large eggs
- 1 cup Extra virgin Olive oil
- 3 large Peeled and chopped Gala apples
- ½ teaspoon Ground cinnamon
- ⅔ cup Gold raisins, soaked and drained
- For dusting purpose confectioner's sugar

Directions

- In a small bowl, soak the gold raisins in lukewarm water for 15 minutes and drain. Keep aside.
- Put the chopped apple in a medium bowl and pour orange juice over it.
- Toss and make sure the apple gets well coated with the orange juice

- Combine cinnamon, flour, baking powder, nutmeg in a large bowl and keep aside.
- Add extra virgin olive oil and sugar into the mixture and combine thoroughly.
- This particular mixture must be thicker in texture and not a runny one.
- In the large bowl that contains the dry ingredients, make a circular path in the middle part of the flour mixture
- Add the olive oil and sugar mixture into this path
- Make use of a wooden spoon and stir them well until they blend well with one another
- It must be a thick batter.
- Drain the excess juice from the apples.
- Add the apples and raisins to the batter and mix it with a spoon to combine.
- Once again, the batter must be reasonably thick in terms of texture.
- In a six-quart slow cooker, place parchment paper and add the batter over it.
- Turn the heat setting to low and the timer to two hours or cook until the cake does not have any wet spots over it
- Once the cake has cooked well, wait until the cake cools down before cutting them into pieces
- Transfer the cake to a serving dish and sprinkle the confectioner's sugar on top.

Mediterranean Crockpot Strawberry Basil Cobbler

7 Servings

Preparation Time: 2 hours 50 minutes

Ingredients

- ½ cup Skim milk
- 3 Eggs
- ¼ teaspoon Divided salt
- 4 tablespoons Canola oil
- ¼ cup Rolled oats
- 6 cups frozen strawberries
- 3 cups Vanilla frozen yogurt
- ¼ cup Chopped fresh basil
- 1¼ cups Divided granulated sugar
- 2½ cups Divided whole wheat flour
- ½ teaspoon Ground cinnamon
- 2 teaspoons Baking powder
- Cooking spray

Directions

- Combine sugar, flour, baking powder, salt and cinnamon in a large bowl.

- Add the milk, oil, and eggs into the bowl and combine thoroughly.
- Coat some olive oil in the bottom of the slow cooker.
- Transfer and spread the mixed batter evenly into the slow cooker.
- Take another large bowl and combine flour, salt, and sugar.
- Add basil and strawberries to the bowl and toss it to coat.
- Pour this mixture on the top of the batter in the slow cooker.
- Top up with the rolled oat mixture.
- Close the slow cooker and cook on a high heat setting for 2½ hours. You can check the cooking status by inserting a toothpick. If it comes out clean, your cake is ready.
- Serve topped with frozen vanilla yogurt and basil.

Slow Cooker Mediterranean Pumpkin Pecan Bread Pudding

5 Servings

Preparation Time: 4 hours15 minutes

Ingredients

- 1 cup canned pumpkin
- ½ cup Melted butter
- ½ cup Brown sugar
- ½ teaspoon Cinnamon
- 1 teaspoon Vanilla
- ¼ teaspoon Ground ginger
- ½ teaspoon Nutmeg
- ¼ cup Vanilla ice cream
- ½ cup Chopped toasted pecans
- 8 cups Day-old whole wheat bread cubes
- 4 Eggs
- ½ cup Cinnamon chips
- 1 cup Half n half
- ⅛ teaspoon Ground cloves
- ¼ cup Caramel ice cream topping

Directions

- Grease a 6-quart crockpot and put the bread cubes, cinnamon, and chopped pecans into it.
- In a medium bowl, whisk together pumpkin, eggs, brown sugar, half-n-half, vanilla, melted butter, nutmeg, cinnamon, cloves, ginger and pour the mixture over the bread cubes.
- Stir the mix gently.
- Cover up the slow cooker and cook for 4 hours. It will be well prepared within 4 hours.
- Before serving, top up with caramel ice cream and vanilla ice cream.

Slow Cooker Chocolate Fondue

5 Servings

Preparation Time: 2 hours15 minutes

Ingredients

- 1½ tablespoons Butter
- 3 tablespoons Milk
- 1½ cups Miniature marshmallows
- 4½ ounces Chocolate Almonds candy bars
- ½ cup Heavy whipping cream

Directions

- Grease a 2-quart slow cooker and put chocolate, butter, milk, marshmallows into it.
- Close the cooker and cook on a low heat setting for 1½ hours.
- Stir the mix every 30 minutes to melt and mix whipping cream gradually.
- After adding whipping cream, allow it to settle for 2 hours.
- Use it as a chocolate dip.

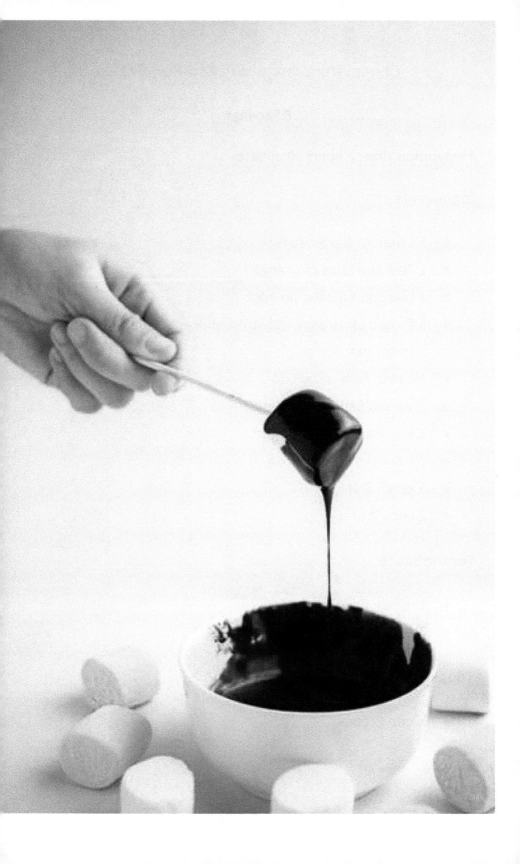

Chocolate Orange Volcano Pudding

8 Servings

Preparation Time: 2 hours 20 minutes

Ingredients

- 5¼ ounces Caster sugar
- 1 Zest and juice of orange
- 1 teaspoon Baking powder
- 5¼ ounces orange flavored milk chocolate, chopped into chunks
- 1½ cups Milk
- ½ pound Self-raising flour
- 3½ ounces Melted butter
- 2¾ ounces Sifted cocoa
- A pinch Salt
- 2 cups Water

For the Sauce

- 1 ounce Cocoa
- 7½ ounces Light brown soft sugar

Topping

- ¼ cup Cream

- ¼ cup Vanilla ice cream
- 1 Orange wedges

Directions

- Grease the slow cooker with butter.
- Combine the caster sugar, flour, baking powder, and cocoa, pinch of salt, and orange zest in a large mixing bowl thoroughly.
- Whisk the eggs, orange juice, milk, and buttermilk in a medium bowl.
- Add it to the dry ingredients and combine to form a smooth mixture.
- Stir in chocolate pieces and then transfer the mixture into the slow cooker
- Prepare the sauce by mixing cocoa and sugar in two cups of boiling water.
- Pour the sauce over the pudding mixture.
- Cover the slow cooker and cook on high heat for two hours.
- Before serving, top the pudding with vanilla ice cream or cream and orange wedges.

Slow Cooker Nutella Fudge

7 Servings

Preparation Time: 1 hour 40 minutes

Ingredients

- 7 0unces 70 percent dark chocolate
- 1 cup Nutella
- 4 ounces Chopped toasted hazelnuts
- 1 teaspoon Vanilla essence
- 14 ounces Condensed milk
- 3 ounces Icing sugar

Directions

- In a slow cooker, add vanilla essence, condensed milk, dark chocolate, and Nutella.
- Cook it for 1½ hours without covering the lid.
- Make sure to stir the ingredients every ten minutes until they melt completely.
- After cooking, turn off the slow cooker and transfer its content into a large-sized mixing bowl
- Stir in the sieved icing sugar.
- Take the warm fudge and carefully scrape it flat, and allow it cool.

- Sprinkle the hazelnuts over the fudge and slightly press them downwards so that they get attached well.
- Refrigerate this well for 4 hours and then cut them into squares.

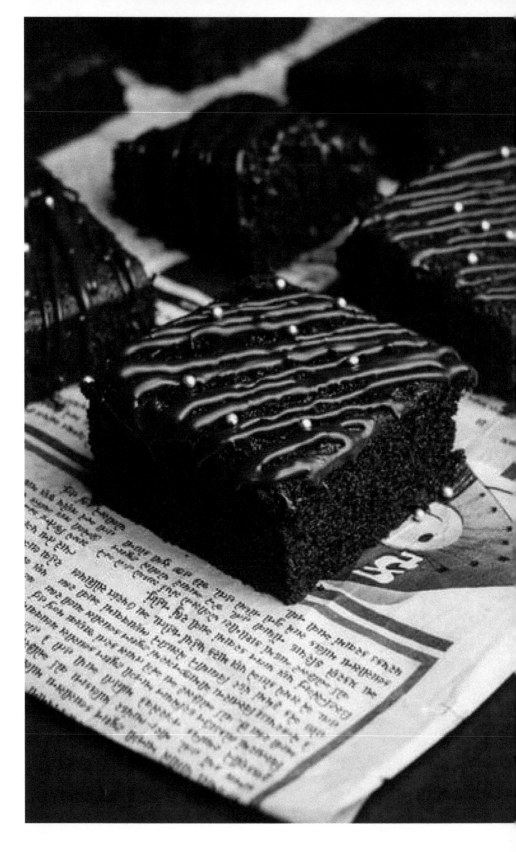

Greek Yogurt Chocolate Mousse

6 Servings

Preparation Time: 2 hours 5 minutes

Ingredients

- ¾ cup Milk
- 1 tablespoon Maple syrup
- 2 cups Greek yogurt
- 3½ ounces Dark chocolate
- ½ teaspoon Vanilla extract

Directions

- Pour milk into a glass bowl that can be placed inside the slow cooker.
- Add the chocolate, either as finely chopped or as a grated one, into the glass bowl.
- Place the bowl inside the slow cooker.
- Pour water surrounding the bowl.
- Cook it for 2 hours on low heat by stirring intermittently.
- Once the chocolate is combined thoroughly with the milk, turn off the cooker and remove the glass bowl from the slow cooker.

- Add vanilla extract and maple syrup to the bowl and stir well.
- Spoon in the Greek yogurt in a large bowl and add the chocolate mixture on top of it.
- Mix it well together before serving.
- Refrigerate for two hours before serving.

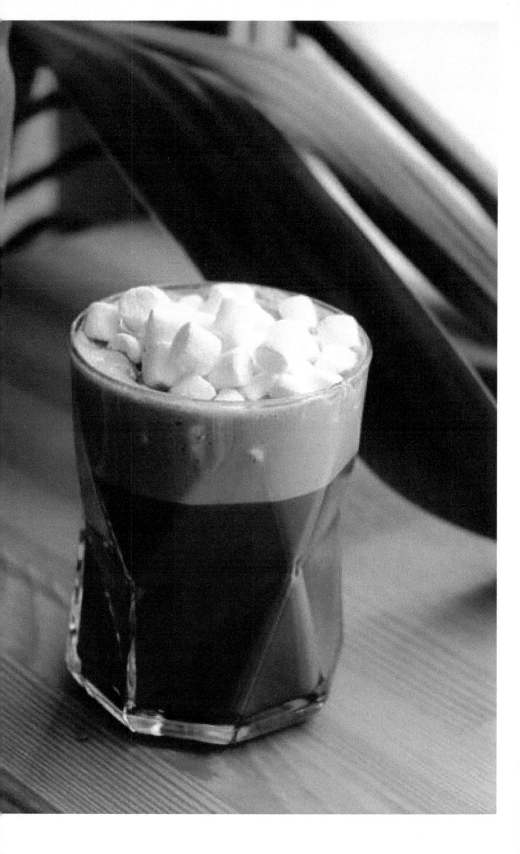

Peanut Butter Banana Greek Yogurt Bowl

6 Servings

Preparation Time: 2 hours5 minutes

Ingredients

- 4 cups Vanilla Greek yogurt

- ¼ cup Flaxseed meal

- ¼ cup Creamy natural peanut butter

- 3 Sliced bananas

- 1 teaspoon Nutmeg

Directions

- Divide the yogurt between four different bowls and top it with banana slices.

- Add peanut butter into a small-sized glass bowl and place in the slow cooker.

- Pour water surrounding the glass bowl.

- Under a low heat setting, cook without covering the slow cooker until the peanut butter starts to melt.

- The peanut butter should be in a thick consistency.

- Once the butter turns to the required consistency, remove the bowl from the slow cooker.

- Now, scoop one tablespoon of melted peanut butter and serve into the bowl with yogurt and bananas.

- For each bowl, add about one tablespoon of melted peanut butter.

- Sprinkle ground nutmeg and flaxseed.

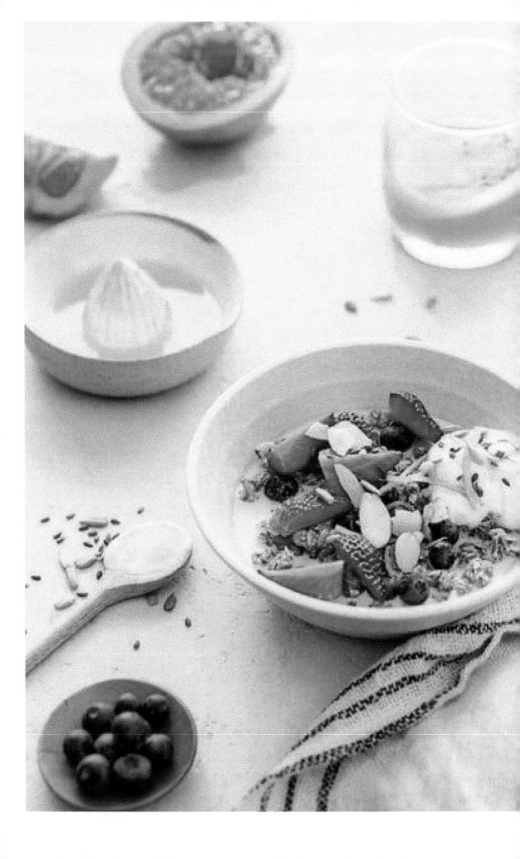

Italian Slow Cooker Banana Foster

6 Servings

Preparation Time: 2 hours10 minutes

Ingredients

- ¼ cup Rum
- 1 cup Brown sugar
- ½ teaspoon Cinnamon, ground
- 1 teaspoon Vanilla extract
- 6 Bananas
- 4 tablespoons Butter, melted
- ¼ cup Coconut, shredded
- ¼ cup Walnuts, chopped

Directions

- Peel the bananas, slice and keep ready to use.
- Place the sliced bananas in the slow cooker in layers.
- Mix the brown sugar, vanilla, butter, rum and cinnamon in a medium bowl thoroughly.
- Pour the mix over the bananas.
- Close the slow cooker and cook on low heat for 2 hours.
- Sprinkle shredded coconut and walnuts on top before 30 of the end process, and serve.

Melon Pudding

3 Servings

Preparation time: 10 minutes 3 hours

Ingredients

- 1 cup melon, chopped
- 2 tablespoons cornstarch
- 1 teaspoon vanilla extract
- ¼ cup of coconut milk

Direction

- Blend the melon until smooth and mix with coconut milk, cornstarch, and vanilla extract.
- Transfer the mixture into the slow cooker and cook the pudding on Low for 3 hours.

Stuffed Peaches

4 Servings

Preparation time: 15 minutes 20 minutes

Ingredients

- 1 tablespoon maple syrup
- 2 oz goat cheese, crumbled
- 4 peaches, halved, pitted
- 4 pecans

Direction

- Fill every peach half with pecan and sprinkle with maple syrup.
- Then put the fruits in the slow cooker in one layer and top with goat cheese.
- Close the lid and cook the peaches for 20 minutes on High.

Sponge Cake

6 Servings

Preparation time: 15 minutes 7 hours

Ingredients

- 1 cup of sugar
- ½ cup flour
- 1 teaspoon vanilla extract
- Cooking spray
- 2 egg yolks
- 4 egg whites

Direction

- Spray the slow cooker with cooking spray from inside.
- Then whisk the egg whites until you get soft peaks.
- After this, mix egg yolks with sugar and blend until smooth.
- Add flour and vanilla extract.
- Then add egg whites and carefully mix the mixture until homogenous.
- Pour it in the slow cooker and close the lid.
- Cook the sponge cake on Low for 7 hours.

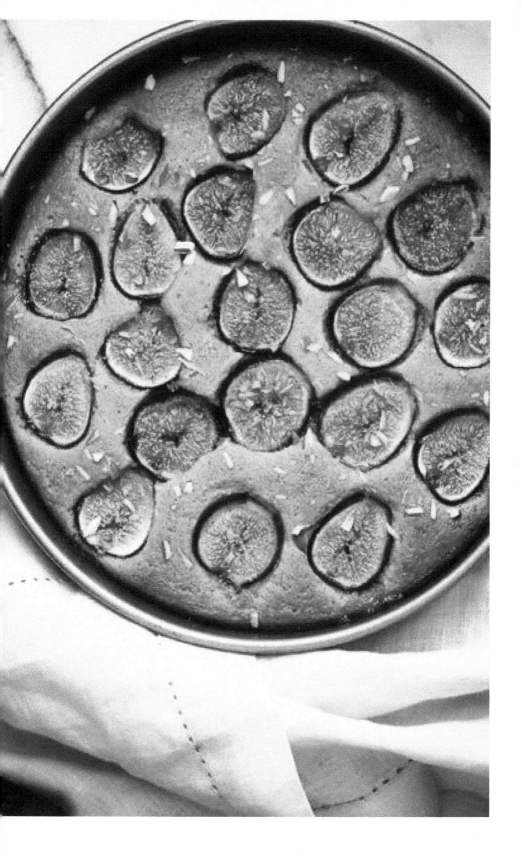

Semolina Pie

4 Servings

Preparation time10 minutes 2 hours

Ingredients

- ½ cup cottage cheese
- 1 tablespoon flour
- ½ cup semolina
- 2 tablespoons butter, melted
- 1 teaspoon vanilla extract
- 1 teaspoon corn starch

Direction

- Mix semolina with cottage cheese and vanilla extract.
- Then add corn starch, flour, and butter.
- Blend the mixture with the help of the blender until smooth and put in the slow cooker. Flatten it.
- Close the lid and cook the semolina pie for 2 hours on High.

SOUP AND STEW

Fennel Stew

6 servings

Preparation time: 15 minutes, 5 hours

Ingredients

- 1-pound beef sirloin, chopped
- 1 tablespoon dried dill
- 1 teaspoon olive oil
- 1 cup fennel bulb, chopped
- 3 cups of water
- 1 yellow onion, chopped

Direction

- Roast the beef sirloin in the skillet for 2 minutes per side.
- Then transfer the meat in the slow cooker.
- Add olive oil, a fennel bulb, water, onion, and dried dill.
- Close the lid and cook the stew on high for 5 hours.

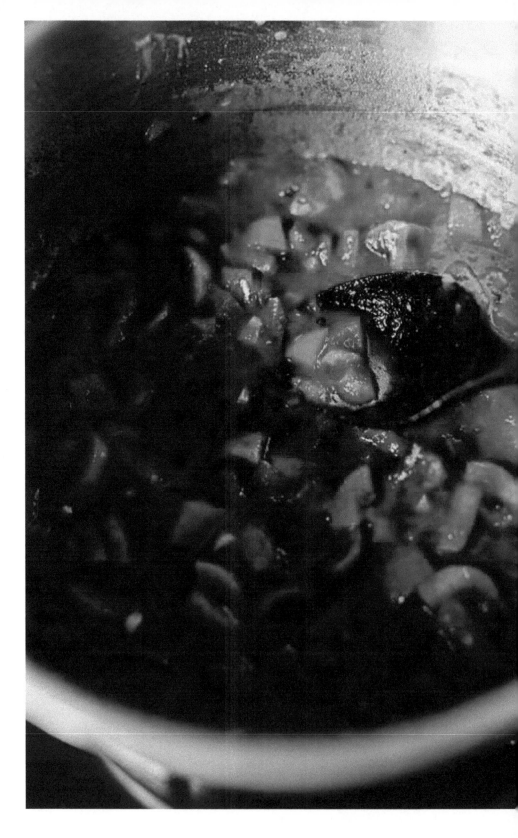

Cabbage Stew

2 Servings

Preparation time: 7 minutes 3 hours

Ingredients

- 2 cups white cabbage, shredded
- ½ cup tomato juice
- 1 teaspoon ground white pepper
- 1 cup cauliflower, chopped
- ½ cup potato, chopped
- 1 cup of water

Direction

- Put cabbage, potato, and cauliflower in the slow cooker.
- Add tomato juice, ground white pepper, and water. Stir the stew ingredients and close the lid.
- Cook the stew on high for 3 hours.

Smoked Sausage Stew

5 Servings

Preparation time: 10 minutes 3.5 hours

Ingredients

- 1-pound smoked sausages, chopped
- 1 teaspoon butter
- 1 teaspoon dried thyme
- ¼ cup Cheddar cheese, shredded
- 1 cup broccoli, chopped
- 1 cup tomato juice
- 1 cup of water

Direction

- Grease the slow cooker bowl with butter from inside.
- Put the smoked sausages in one layer in the slow cooker.
- Add the layer of broccoli and Cheddar cheese.
- Then mix water with tomato juice and dried thyme.
- Pour the liquid over the sausage mixture and close the lid.
- Cook the stew on high for 3.5 hours.

Meat Baby Carrot Stew

3 Servings

Preparation time: 10 minutes 8 hours

Ingredients

- 1 cup baby carrot
- 1 teaspoon peppercorns
- 3 cups of water
- 1 bay leaf
- 6 oz lamb loin, chopped
- 1 tablespoon tomato paste

Direction

- Put all ingredients in the slow cooker.
- Close the lid and cook the stew on Low for 8 hours.
- Carefully stir the stew and cool it to room temperature.

Jamaican Stew

8 Servings

Preparation time: 15 minutes 1 hour

Ingredients

- 1-pound salmon fillet, chopped
- 1 teaspoon ground coriander
- ½ teaspoon ground cumin
- 1 tablespoon coconut oil
- 1 teaspoon garlic powder
- ½ cup bell pepper, sliced
- ½ cup heavy cream

Direction

- Put the coconut oil in the slow cooker.
- Then mix the salmon with ground cumin and ground coriander and put in the slow cooker.
- Add the layer of bell pepper and sprinkle with garlic powder.
- Add heavy cream and close the lid.
- Cook the stew on High for 1 hour.

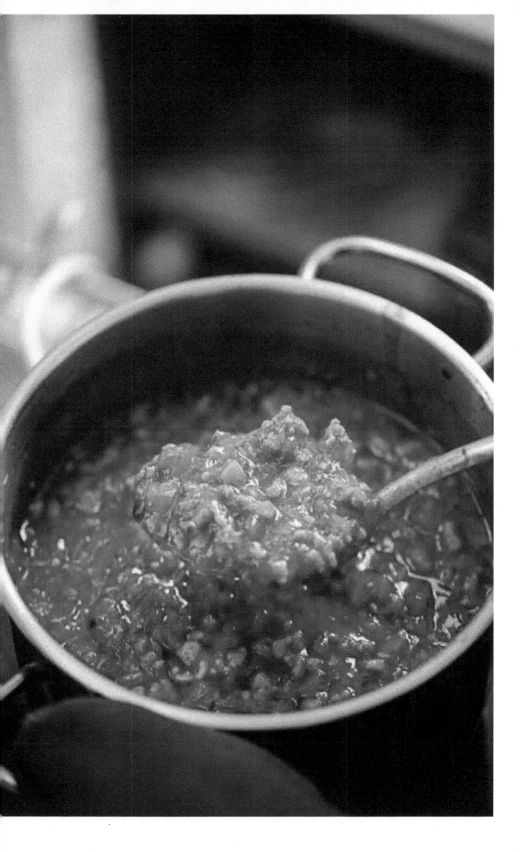